PCOS

COOKBOOK

65 Recipes

Iduna Dietitian

Table of Contents

Other dishes

Salads

Desserts

3-days menu

INTRODUCTION

Lack of periods, hirsutism, acne, bad mood, and extra pounds. Unfortunately, if you have this combination of symptoms, you probably have polycystic ovarian syndrome (PCOS).

Polycystic ovarian syndrome is the most common endocrine disorder found in women of childbearing age. It has been shown to affect up to 5-20% of premenopausal women. Fortunately, PCOS can also be successfully treated with diet.

Dunaif A, Hyperandrogenic anovulation (PCOS): A unique disorder of insulin action associated with an increased risk of non-insulin-dependent diabetes mellitus. The American Journal of Medicine, 1995, 98(1), S33-S39

With this book:
- you will learn what to eat to improve your health, what foods will help you fight the negative effects, what to avoid in PCOS, and how to prepare meals,
- you will learn what kind of supplementation will bring positive effects,
- you will learn 65 different recipes for delicious sweets and cakes, savory dinners and appetizers, original salads, unique soups,
- you will receive a 3-day balanced menu containing all the essential nutrients that our body needs to function properly.

PCOS

PCOS, polycystic ovary syndrome is the most common endocrine disorder among women of childbearing age, and according to various data, 5 to 20% of women of childbearing age may suffer from the disease.

In most cases, PCOS is associated with excess body weight, insulin resistance, disturbances in the lipid profile (cholesterol and triglycerides), and, consequently, an increased risk of cardiovascular disease. That is why it is so important to introduce eating habits quickly enough, without waiting for symptoms or complications to appear.

DIAGNOSIS OF PCOS

The diagnosis is always made by a doctor: an endocrinologist or a gynecologist. According to the Rotterdam Criteria adopted in 2004, the diagnosis of PCOS requires the presence of two out of three symptoms:

- Menstrual disorders (of any kind, whether associated with too long or too short cycles, with excessive or no bleeding)
- Clinical or biochemical symptoms of excess male sex hormones (androgens). It can be manifested by persistent acne, excessively oily skin, characteristic alopecia areata, or the appearance of hair typical of men (hirsutism),
- The presence of ovarian cysts visible on the transvaginal ultrasound image (always interpreted by a specialist).

In contrast, the 2006 Androgen Excess and PCOS Society criteria require the presence of hyperandrogenism for diagnosis, which creates confusion in the diagnosis of PCOS. Many of the above-mentioned symptoms accompany other diseases, so the specialist always excludes possible causes of the above disorders, referring us to additional tests.

We should never do them on our own because there are no laboratory tests that would clearly confirm Polycystic Ovary Syndrome. Diagnosis is largely based on an interview, which must always be performed by a specialist.

SYMPTOMS OF PCOS

This disease contributes to the occurrence of metabolic disorders, primarily **insulin resistance**, and consequently **obesity**, and an increased risk of **type 2 diabetes**. That is why diet is so important in this disorder. You may also experience problems with **mental malaise**, **acne**, and **infertility**.

A proper diet combined with physical activity will not only help in the fight against unnecessary kilograms and improve tissue sensitivity to insulin, but also improve blood parameters, and very often it can also have a positive effect on the fertility of a woman with PCOS.

Symptoms :

- lengthening menstrual cycles,
- difficulties in getting pregnant
- symptoms related to excess androgens:
    - hirsutism, or excessive,
    - body hair,
    - persistent acne,
    - alopecia,
    - uncontrolled weight gain.

CONSEQUENCES OF UNTREATED PCOS

PCOS is not only an ovarian disease and an infertility problem. Untreated polycystic ovary syndrome also has an impact on long-term health effects. From an increased risk of metabolic diseases to severe mood swings and depression, to ovarian and uterine cancer.

WHY PCOS?

Both your genes and environmental factors are responsible for the occurrence of PCOS. For example, there is a close relationship between PCOS and obesity. Up to 90% of women with PCOS also have obesity. On the one hand, PCOS increases the risk of obesity, and on the other hand, obesity increases the negative consequences of PCOS.

What do PCOS and obesity have in common? Insulin resistance (IO). It's actually a kind of PCOS litmus test. Even if your body weight is normal, but your genes have beaten you PCOS, you are likely to have IO.

Legro, Richard S., 2012, Obesity and PCOS: implications for diagnosis and treatment." Seminars in reproductive medicine. Vol. 30. No. 6. NIH Public Access.

Insulin stimulates the production of androgens ("male" hormones) in the body. Increased insulin levels also inhibit the production of the testosterone transport protein (SHBG), which results in increased hyperandrogenism (more available testosterone circulates in the blood). If we add obesity to it, which exacerbates the problem of IO, all the consequences of PCOS become stronger.

Azziz, Ricardo, 2018, Polycystic ovary syndrome, Obstetrics & Gynecology 132.2, 321-336.

DIET IN PCOS

How diet can help you:
- balance insulin levels, which improves insulin sensitivity,
- reducing symptoms of hyperandrogenism - acne, hair loss,
- restoring regular ovulation.

What can help you:

- low glycemic index foods,
- Mediterranean diet,
- antioxidants,
- Omega-3 fatty acids,
- adequate levels of vitamin D, zinc, and selenium,
- avoiding processed foods and sources of trans fats,
- proper heat processing of prepared foods.

The most important dietary goal in PCOS is to achieve a **normal body weight** - even a few percent reductions in excess weight have beneficial health effects, such as:
- improving lipid and glucose parameters,
- may restore regular menstrual periods
- significantly increase the chances of having children.

Barber, Thomas M., et al. (2019), Obesity and polycystic ovary syndrome: implications for pathogenesis and novel management strategies, Clinical Medicine Insights: Reproductive Health 13, 1179558119874042

The first step is to realize how much energy we need in general.

You don't need to know complicated formulas to calculate such a demand.

You can use this special calculator.

First, you enter your age, weight, and height, then select the appropriate physical activity.

You have a variety of activity levels to choose: ranging from very low activity to very active people.

The choice is not always clear-cut. It is important to choose the option that is most closely related to our daily activities.

In my experience, if you are wondering which option to choose, the best option is to choose less activity.

After you enter all the necessary parameters, you get the result.

How to read all these numbers?

The first result we get is Maintain weight, which is our requirement. This is the number of calories we should consume during the day to maintain our current body weight. - If your body weight is normal choose this option.

Below the next three results show the calorie value that will make you lose weight.

What caloric value to choose?

If you are overweight or obese, I suggest you choose a weight loss that is about 0.5 kg/week.

Each recipe in this book has a calorie listed, which can help you stick to a certain calorie throughout the day.

For example, if your caloric requirement is 1500 kcal then you can use:

- Breakfast: Bounty balls - 439 kcal
- Lunch: Peppers stuffed with quinoa and vegetables - 397 kcal
- Snack: Sandwiches with avocado paste - 302
- Supper: Quinoa with raspberries - 367 kcal

That's a total of 1505 kcal

Insulin resistance

Insulin resistance is a metabolic condition in which tissue sensitivity to insulin is reduced.

And what does insulin do?

- causes glycogen deposition in the liver and skeletal muscles,
- increases amino acid uptake by tissues and enhances protein synthesis,
- stimulates the formation of fatty acids and inhibits their breakdown, which leads to the storage of free fatty acids in the form of triacylglycerols in adipose tissue,
- increases the uptake of amino acids by tissues and enhances protein synthesis,
- is a hormone that lowers blood glucose levels by increasing glucose uptake by muscle and adipose tissue,
- stimulates glucose storage in the form of glycogen in muscle and liver.

Deteriorating insulin sensitivity forces pancreatic cells to produce more insulin. Insulin must do its job, otherwise, there would be too much glucose circulating in our blood, but if tissues are resistant to insulin, despite adequate blood levels, the body tries to cope by increasing the production of the hormone.

When adipose tissue loses its ability to store energy in the form of fat, large amounts of free fatty acids are released from it, and it also becomes a source of pro-inflammatory cytokines that activate inflammation.

Dietary causes of insulin resistance:

inappropriate diet over a long period of time:

- rich in simple sugars and saturated fats.
- processed and low in nutrients.
- high amounts of sweets, fast food, processed meat
- foods in batter, with roux, fried foods, and thick, fatty sauces.

Neglected insulin resistance in the long term can progress to type 2 diabetes.

A diet that improves insulin sensitivity, thereby helping to regulate sex hormone levels and consequently reducing symptoms, is characterized by:

- low glycemic load,
- high protein content (keeping to recommended norms),
- moderate carbohydrates,
- the presence of regular physical activity - is a very important aspect.

Muscles use about 70% of the glucose circulating in our bodies. If they do not need it, because we have too little physical activity, the excess glucose goes back to the liver. There, fatty acids are formed from glucose, which in a further step contributes to the growth of adipose tissue and deterioration of insulin sensitivity.

Low glycemic index foods

Using the glycemic index is especially important for people who struggle with insulin resistance.

As a result, we are able to control carbohydrate metabolism. This is very important in regulating blood glucose levels and insulin resistance.

The Glycemic index is an index that shows how rapidly blood glucose levels change within 120 minutes of consuming a serving of a product containing 50 grams of assimilable carbohydrates, compared to consuming 50 grams of pure glucose.

The higher the glycemic index value, the faster and higher the blood glucose concentration rises after eating a food, and then it falls quickly (very often below the baseline concentration, which is unfavorable).

It is important for our health that blood sugar levels do not rise too high and too fast at the same time. Therefore, it is believed that we should eat products with a low glycemic index.

Based on the glycemic index value, foods were divided into products with:

- low glycemic index (<50)
- medium glycemic index (51-75)
- large glycemic index (>75)

GLYCEMIC INDEX VALUES

dried spices - 5
onion - 15
zucchini - 15
chicory - 15
blackcurrant - 15
green beans - 15
mushrooms - 15
sprouts (mung beans, soya beans) - 15
sauerkraut - 15
cucumber - 15
olives - 15
nuts and almonds - 15
peppers (red, green, yellow) - 15
leek - 15
celery - 15
soya, tofu - 15
asparagus - 15
green leafy vegetables - 15
eggplant - 20
cherries - 20
lemon juice (unsweetened) - 20
dark chocolate (70% cocoa) - 25
red currant - 25
blueberries - 25
pumpkin seeds - 25
cherries - 25
green lentils - 25
cooked chickpeas - 30

red lentils - 30
garlic - 30
low-sugar jam - 30
pear - 30
chinese noodles - 30
soya milk - 30
fresh apricots - 30
citrus fruits - 30
tomatoes - 30
fat free quark - 30
amaranth - 35
beans - 35
peaches, nectarines - 35
wild rice - 35
green peas - 35
fresh, stewed, dried apples - 35
lowfat yoghurt - 35
mustard - 35
seeds (linseed, sunflower seeds) - 35
sun-dried tomatoes - 35
raw celery (root) - 35
prunes - 35
crisp bread - 35
wholemeal bread and pasta - 40
tinned beans - 40
dried figs - 40
buckwheat groats - 40
al dente pasta - 40
dried apricots, prunes - 40

bran, raw oatmeal - 40
carrot juice - 40
pineapple (fresh) - 45
pearl barley - 45
coconut - 45
brown rice - 45
sugar free citrus juice - 45
grapes - 45
canned green peas - 45
cranberry - 45
spelt bread - 50
kiwi - 50
couscous - 50
basmati rice - 50
sugar free apple juice - 50
surimi (crab sticks) - 50
canned peaches - 55
ketchup - 55
mustard - 55
sugar free grape juice - 55
ripe bananas - 60
sweetened cocoa - 60
sweetened ice cream - 60
mayonnaise - 60
melon - 60
honey - 60
low-fat milk - 60
canned apricots - 60
cooked oatmeal - 60
long grain rice - 60
canned pineapple - 65
cooked beets - 65

jam with sugar - 65
corn - 65
chocolate bars - 65
raisins - 65
jacket potatoes - 65
baguette - 70
sponge cake - 70
wheat rolls - 70
crisps - 70
rice bread - 70
sugar - 70
dried dates - 70
barley groats - 70
rice gruel - 70
white flour pasta - 70
corn flour - 70
sodas - 70
short grain rice - 70
rusks - 70
cooked potatoes - 70
pumpkin, squash - 75
french fries - 75
cooked broad beans - 80
cooked carrots - 80
wheat flour - 85
corn flakes - 82
roasted corn - 85
white flour bread - 90
potato flour - 90
baked potatoes - 95
fried potatoes - 95
beer - 110

It is important to remember that a low index is not everything.

Glycemic load also matters, which takes into account not only the index but also the portion of the product. In this case, it is also important to properly compose whole meals, that is, pay attention to the fact that each of them, even a snack, contains a source of complex carbohydrates, healthy fat, and protein.

A low glycemic load diet is rich in **fiber**.

It is found in vegetables, fruits, and whole grains such as wholemeal bread, oatmeal, groats, and brown rice. It is also characterized by a higher intake of protein and the inclusion of healthy fats such as olive oil, flaxseed oil, nuts, almonds, and seeds.

What affects GI:

- particle size - the more fragmented the product, the higher the GI, for example, oatmeal will be a better choice than semolina or fruit whole than in a smoothie or juice,
- the degree of gelatinization of the starch (basically the degree of overcooking) - the more water-soaked the starch, the higher the GI. Kasha cooked al'dente will be a better choice than overcooked,
- the addition of fat and protein - fat has a GI = 0, and protein delays gastric emptying, so its addition will lower the GI of the dish. A balanced meal (containing both carbohydrates, fat, protein, and vegetables) is a much better choice than one containing almost only carbohydrates (e.g. pasta with strawberries),
- fiber content - the addition of fiber makes the product take longer to digest and therefore has a lower GI. Choose coarse groats (buckwheat, pearl barley, bulgur) and wholemeal bread instead of white bread and fine groats (e.g. couscous, semolina),

Mediterranean diet

It is a model of nutrition-based primarily on healthy eating habits.

The principles of the Mediterranean diet:
- Relying on unprocessed, natural products,
- reducing consumption of red meat in favor of fish and legumes as sources of protein,
- eating lots of fruits and vegetables rich in antioxidants,
- using olive oil as the main source of supplemental fats,
- eating whole grain products - bread, rice, pasta, groats,
- replace salt with herbs - salt can be pro-inflammatory and can aggravate acne. This includes salt added to meals as well as highly processed foods that contain large amounts of salt.

A study of 75 women following the Mediterranean diet found that these women lost an average of 6.3 pounds in 12 weeks (this was also the result of a calorie deficit, not the diet itself). Total cholesterol and LDL cholesterol levels also decreased significantly, while HDL cholesterol levels increased (a welcome change). Free testosterone levels also decreased, while SHBG levels increased. Inflammatory markers also decreased - CRP by 35% and SAA by 38%.

Moran LJ, Grieger JA, Mishra GD, Teede HJ. (2015) The Association of a Mediterranean-Style Diet Pattern with Polycystic Ovary Syndrome Status in a Community Cohort Study. Nutrients. 2015;7(10):8553-8564

A diet rich in antioxidant sources

In PCOS, there is increased oxidative stress due to higher concentrations of free radicals in the body than in healthy individuals. These radicals react with cellular components, including DNA, and may contribute to metabolic diseases and increase the risk of certain cancers, among other things.

Antioxidants help to reduce the concentration of free radicals. Their sources are mainly fresh vegetables and fruits, nuts, spices, and herbs.

Green tea

Green tea (Camellia sinensis) belongs to the richest plant sources of flavonoids, a group of antioxidants. Its fresh leaves contain a high concentration of catechins, whose therapeutic effect has been proven in the treatment of numerous diseases.

In addition to the effect of lowering insulin and fasting glucose levels, properties such as reducing the risk of cardiovascular disease and metabolic syndrome have been discovered.

For PCOS, the most important properties of green tea are its effects on lowering fasting insulin levels and free testosterone levels.

Turmeric

Turmeric is a very good source of antioxidant curcumin, whose properties are useful in treating PCOS.

What curcumin affects:
- estrogenic and hypoglycemic effects,
- preventing ovarian cell dysfunction,
- alleviating oxidative stress,
- significantly lowering serum triglycerides, total cholesterol, and LDL fractions,
- increase the concentration of HDL fraction cholesterol.

Cinnamon

Cinnamon is known as a medicinal plant, increasing serum progesterone levels during the luteal phase, which helps regulate the menstrual cycle. It also has anti-inflammatory, antioxidant, anti-diabetic, and lipid-lowering properties.

Cinnamon can be added to oatmeal, yogurt, and pancakes, which will lower the glycemic index of the dish and affects the slower release of glucose in the blood.

Omega-3 fatty acids

Omega-3 fatty acids play one the key roles when it comes to improving health in polycystic ovary syndrome.

Omega-3 fatty acids:
- reduce inflammation in the body that accompanies PCOS,
- reduce the risk of metabolic syndrome (hypertension, type 2 diabetes, high triglycerides,
- improve the body's lipid metabolism and the regularity of the monthly cycle,
- contribute to improved insulin sensitivity,
- have a positive effect on the nervous system, which reduces the risk of depression,
- increase the concentration of adiponectin - a hormone produced in adipose tissue, improving the insulin sensitivity of tissues.

Best sources of omega-3:
- flaxseed oil
- linseed
- walnuts
- fish: salmon, mackerel, trout
- cod liver oil

Vitamin D

The deficiency of this vitamin affects the dysfunction of all body systems. It is also suggested that its deficiency is associated with PCOS symptoms, such as insulin resistance, hirsutism, and infertility.

There is a close correlation between vitamin D deficiency and disorders of the monthly cycle and insulin resistance. It has been shown that women with diagnosed PCOS have lower serum levels of this vitamin. Studies have confirmed the effect of vitamin D use on increasing tissue insulin sensitivity.

The particularly beneficial effect of this vitamin in the context of pre-diabetic states is abnormal fasting glucose levels or abnormal glucose tolerance.

Vitamin D deficiency in women with diagnosed PCOS has been shown to correlate with lipid metabolism abnormalities (abnormal total cholesterol and LDL cholesterol levels) or elevated HOMA-IR index.

Wang, L. Wen, X. Li, F. et all. (2020) Vitamin D deficiency is associated with metabolic risk factors in women with polycystic ovary syndrome: a cross- sectional study in Shaanxi- China. Front Endocrinol (Lausanne) 11, 171

Zinc

Zinc is a trace element that plays an important role in many biochemical processes occurring in the human body, including those related to gene expression and stabilization, and cell growth and division.

Moreover, zinc acts as an antioxidant responsible for neutralizing one form of free oxygen radicals.

It is also necessary for the development and proper functioning of the immune system.

Zinc deficiency is characterized by many symptoms, and one of the consequences is reduced glucose tolerance.

In one study in which 220 mg of zinc sulfate (50 mg zinc content) was administered for 8 weeks, a decrease in fasting glucose, and insulin, a decrease in HOMA-IR and HOMA-B indices, and an increase in QUICKI index were observed. A decrease in VLDL cholesterol was also noted.

Foroozanfard, F. Jamilian, M. Jafari, Z.et all. (2015) Effects of zinc supplementation on markers of insulin resistance and lipid profiles in women with polycystic ovary syndrome: a randomized, double-blind, placebo-controlled trial. Exp Clin Endocrinol Diabetes.123(4), 215-20

Sources of zinc in the diet:
- whole grain products- bread, groats
- pulses: lentils, beans, peas, soybeans
- amaranth
- oatmeal
- offal
- eggs
- dairy products
- nuts: walnuts, peanuts, almonds
- shitake mushrooms
- cocoa

Selenium

Selenium is a trace element that participates in many biochemical pathways necessary for the proper functioning of the body. Selenium is also involved in scavenging reactive oxygen species.

Sources of selenium in the diet:
- Brazil nuts,
- poultry,
- eggs,
- dairy products,
- fish - mainly salmon and tuna,
- brassica and onion vegetables,
- cereals,
- legumes,
- asparagus.

Selenium is found in soil and water, so its content in food is highly dependent on the environment.

As an example of Brazil nuts, depending on the country of origin, selenium content varies from 1.6 to 20.2 mcg/g product. The highest amount of selenium was in nuts that came from South America. To supply 100% of an adult's selenium needs, it is enough to consume 2 Brazil nuts that originated in Peru or 4 that originated in Brazil.

A study in which women supplemented selenium at 200 µg daily for 8 weeks showed an effect on insulin regulation and increased insulin sensitivity. A reduction in triglycerides (TG) and VLDL cholesterol levels were also observed.

Jamilian, M. Maryamalsadat, R. Zohren Fakhrie, K. et all. (2015) Metabolic response to selenium supplementation in women with polycystic ovary syndrome: a randomized, double-blind, placebo-controlled trial. Clin Endocrinol (Oxf). 82(6), 885-91

Avoiding processed foods and sources of trans fats

It is very important in the diet for PCOS to avoid highly processed foods, sweets, salty and sugary snacks, and fast foods.

Eliminating these foods will also make it easier to lose weight.

Proper heat treatment of the products being prepared.

How you prepare your meals is also important.

- avoid frying and grilling,
- baking is allowed but without fat,
- boiling in water or steaming is highly recommended.

SUPPLEMENTATION

Inositol

Inositol is an organic compound that can be produced in our bodies. It is also found naturally in some foods, such as grapefruit and other citrus fruits. We provide about 1g of inositol daily with our diet.

The effects of inositol include:

- reducing the degree of insulin resistance,
- reducing LH production,
- reducing prolactin,
- improved LH/FSH ratio,
- helps restore regular ovulation and menstruation,
- reduces the risk of metabolic diseases such as type II diabetes.

Remember to consult your doctor when choosing a supplement so that together you can choose the right one for you.

Vitamin D

Daily supplementation of 2000 IU (50 µg) is recommended for the population of healthy adults up to 75 years of age.

It should be remembered that it is necessary to check the actual level of vitamin D in serum before deciding on the dose of supplementation and that too high a concentration of vitamin D is toxic, so supplementation should be carried out carefully.

Omega-3 fatty acids

Consider supplementation of omega-3 fatty acids in the form of cod liver oil or, for those on a plant-based diet, acids derived from marine algae.

Folic acid

If you are planning to become pregnant, folic acid supplementation is recommended at least 3 months before the planned pregnancy and during the pregnancy.

Folic acid deficiency during this period has negative effects on the baby's nervous system.

According to the RDA, women of childbearing age should take 400 µg of folate daily, and during pregnancy, the supply should increase to 600 µg.

PHYSICAL ACTIVITY

Any physical activity affects health and is helpful to restore normal body weight.

Physical activity is really a great weapon we can use to target PCOS. It makes the tissues more sensitive to insulin, so they need less of it. We can look at this as a bonus so that we can better combat the tissue insulin resistance present in PCOS.

If you are not enthusiastic about physical activity, you can start with small activities for example walking or marching.

Physical activity that you enjoy will be best. It will bring the best results because you will not be forcing yourself to do it.

Physical activity combined with a proper diet, in any case, has benefits and helps reduce body weight.

PLANT-BASED DIET IN PCOS

Plant-based protein sources

In one study, 60 women suffering from the disorder were divided into two groups. The first followed a healthy, balanced Therapeutic Lifestyle Changes (TLC) diet in which protein came primarily from low-fat dairy products and lean meats. The other followed a similar dietary pattern, with two meals replaced with meals in which legumes were the primary source of protein. Both groups were physically active at the time of the study - 5 low-intensity workouts per week. After 4 months, the group consuming more plant-based protein had much more favorable results. Diastolic blood pressure, LDL cholesterol, and triglycerides decreased more than in the TLC group. The area under the insulin response curve in the glucose load test also decreased. There was also an increase in HDL fraction cholesterol (the good one) compared to the TLC group.

Omega-3 fatty acids

Omega-3 fatty acids are very important in PCOS diet therapy.

Plant sources of omega-3:
- flax seeds,
- chia seeds,
- flaxseed oil,
- pumpkin seeds,
- walnuts.

If you are not consuming the above mentioned products it will be beneficial to introduce omega-3 fatty acid supplementation from algae.

Vitamin B12

If you want to follow a plant-based diet, you can't forget about vitamin B12.

The active forms of vitamin B12 are found only in animal products.

The only way for vegans to get this vitamin is through supplementation or consumption of products fortified with this vitamin.

Unfortunately, fortified foods alone are not enough to satisfy the need for vitamin B12.

It is recommended to take 250 mcg daily or 500 mcg once every two days or you can buy a 1000 mcg tablet and take it twice a week.

NORMAL WEIGHT AND PCOS

How to check if my body weight is correct?

In this case, we can also use a ready-made calculator that will calculate the BMI value.

We need to enter our age, height, weight, and gender.

After entering these data, we get the result.

What about your diet?

Normal body weight is not a guarantee of no **insulin resistance**. It occurs in 6-22% of lean women with PCOS.

Even if polycystic ovary syndrome is not accompanied by OI, normal weight women with PCOS often have higher blood insulin levels than those without polycystic ovary syndrome.

Therefore, a **low glycemic index** diet is also advisable for those of us with PCOS who are of normal weight.

The presence of **antioxidants** in the diet of people with PCOS is also important.

Free radicals (i.e. reactive oxygen species) are constantly formed during all metabolic processes occurring in the body. In PCOS, the ability of antioxidants to scavenge free radicals is reduced in the body. Oxidative stress causes damage to all cell components, including DNA.

Olga Papalou & Evanthia Diamanti-Kandarakis (2017) The role of stress in PCOS, Expert Review of Endocrinology & Metabolism, 12:1, 87-95, DOI: 10.1080/17446651.2017.1266250

This is why the diet for polycystic ovary syndrome should be particularly rich in antioxidants found, for example, in fruits and vegetables.

Diet and supplementation are important in reducing the symptoms characteristic of PCOS, such as lowering androgen levels, reducing hirsutism, and returning ovulation regularity.

For example, **myo-inositol** supplementation, in addition to improving insulin sensitivity, results in a decrease in CRP (an indicator of inflammation) and LH hormone, which are often elevated in polycystic ovary syndrome.

SUMMARY

- if you are overweight or obese, use a calorie requirement calculator to find out how many calories you need to reduce your body weight,
- include physical activity in your daily routine,
- base your diet mainly on products with a low glycemic index
- include fish such as salmon, mackerel, and trout in your diet, or supplement omega-3 fatty acids in the form of fish oil or algae,
- avoid processed foods such as cookies, chips, and fast food,
- eat more fruits and vegetables,
- use cinnamon, and turmeric as an addition to your meals
- replace salt with herbs,
- choose whole grain products,
- do not overcook cereals, or rice - this avoids an increase in the glycemic index
- remember to use healthy fats such as linseed oil, olive oil,
- introduce green tea into your diet
- avoid frying and grilling,
- consider introducing legumes into your diet,
- take supplements: inositol, vitamin D,
- if you follow a vegan diet, remember to take a vitamin B12 supplement
- if you are planning pregnancy, include folic acid in your daily supplementation

TIME FOR recipes

Salmon with asparagus

Ingredients

- **Salmon, fresh**: 100 g
- 1 tsp **Lemon juice**: 3 g
- 5 **Asparagus**: 150 g
- 1 tbsp **Linseed oil**: 10 g
- 1 clove **Garlic**: 6 g
- 1 tsp **Dill**: 4 g
- 1 pinch of **dried basil**
- 1 pinch of **black pepper**

Instructions

Preheat the oven to 230 ° C.

Cut the salmon into portions, place on a board with the skin down, and moving the knife along the fillet between the skin and the meat, cut off the skin. Rinse the fillets, pat them dry, season with pepper, and drizzle with lemon juice.

Wash the asparagus, and break off the hard ends (they will break by themselves in the right place). Put it together with the salmon in an ovenproof dish. Add pressed garlic, chopped dill, and basil.

Mix and drizzle oil over the top of the salmon and asparagus.

Place in the oven and bake uncovered for 15 minutes.

Energy: 342 kcal
Protein: 23 g
Fat: 24 g
Carbohydrates: 9 g
Fiber: 4 g
Glycemic index: 18
Glycemic load: 1

Salmon roasted in oranges

Ingredients

- Salmon, fresh: 100 g
- 1/4 Orange: 60
- 1 tbsp Linseed oil: 10 g
- 2 tsp Parsley, leaves: 10 g
- 2 Walnuts: 8 g
- 1 tsp Dried cranberries: 7 g
- 1/3 tsp Grated lemon peel: 1 g
- 1 tsp Lemon juice: 3 g
- 1 pinch of dried rosemary
- 1 pinch of black pepper

Instructions

Preheat the oven to 180 ° C. Wash the salmon and dry
with a paper towel. Sprinkle with freshly ground pepper
on each side. Place in an ovenproof dish. Pour the oil.
Add rosemary. Scrub the orange, cut it into slices, and
cover the salmon with them. Bake the salmon for about
25 minutes in the oven. In the meantime, heat the
frying pan properly. Roast the nuts on it until they
brown and then chop them. Chop the cranberries into
smaller pieces. Mix nuts, cranberries, chopped parsley,
and lemon zest. When the salmon is baked, remove the
rosemary and orange slices from the salmon and serve
them next to it. Put the prepared topping on the
salmon. Drizzle the whole thing with lemon.

Energy: 405 kcal
Protein: 22 g
Fat: 28 g
Carbohydrates: 16 g
Fiber: 3 g
Glycemic index: 34
Glycemic load: 5

Steamed salmon marinated in lemon juice

Ingredients

- **Salmon, fresh**: 100 g
- 3 tbsp **Lemon juice**: 18 g
- 2 tbsp **Buckwheat groats**: 30 g
- 5 leaves **Lettuce**: 25 g
- 3 **Cherry tomato**: 60 g
- 1 tsp **Pumpkin, seeded, shelled**: 5 g
- 1 tsp **Linseed oil**: 5 g
- 1 pinch of **black pepper**
- 1 pinch of **dried marjoram**
- 1 pinch of **dried basil**
- 1 tbsp **Radish, sprouts**: 10 g

PREP TIME: 5 MINUTES
TOTAL TIME: 65 MINUTES

Energy: 424 kcal
Protein: 27 g
Fat: 22 g
Carbohydrates: 30 g
Fiber: 4 g
Glycemic index: 44
Glycemic load: 11

Instructions

Wash the salmon, put it in a bowl, add the lemon juice and spices and marinate for one hour in the refrigerator. Steam the salmon. Cook the buckwheat groats al dente. Rinse the lettuce under running water, and dry. Put into a bowl. Wash cherry tomatoes, cut in half, and add to the salad, mix with pumpkin seeds, pour a teaspoon of flax oil, and sprinkle with sprouts.

Salmon in stewed tomatoes

Ingredients

PREP TIME: 5 MINUTES
TOTAL TIME: 35 MINUTES

- **Salmon, fresh**: 100 g
- 1 **Tomato**: 160 g
- 1/4 **Lemon**: 22 g
- 3 slices **Onion**: 24 g
- 5 leaves **Basil, fresh**: 5 g

Instructions

Clean and rinse the salmon fillet. Make a marinade from chopped dill and lemon juice, pour it over the fish, and set it aside in the fridge. Dice the onion and tomatoes, put them in a bowl, add chopped basil, and mix. Steam the prepared vegetable mixture in a stacked pot, after 15 minutes place the salmon pieces and steam for another 15 minutes. Put the salmon pieces on a plate, mix the vegetables and serve the fish with the sauce.

Energy: 250 kcal
Protein: 22 g
Fat: 14 g
Carbohydrates: 10 g
Fiber: 3 g
Glycemic index: 24
Glycemic load: 1

Salmon in peanut brittle

Ingredients

PREP TIME: 10 MINUTES
TOTAL TIME: 75 MINUTES

- **Salmon, fresh**: 100 g
- 2 tbsp **Parsley, leaves**: 20 g
- 4 **Walnuts**: 16 g
- 1 tsp **Lemon juice**: 3 g
- 1 pinch of **dried basil**
- 1 pinch of **black pepper**

Instructions

Rub the salmon with basil, and pepper, drizzle with lemon juice and top with parsley. Set aside in the fridge for 45 minutes. Place in an ovenproof dish and sprinkle with ground nuts. Bake for about 20 minutes in an oven preheated to 180 ° C.

Energy: 327 kcal
Protein: 24 g
Fat: 24 g
Carbohydrates: 6 g
Fiber: 3 g
Glycemic index: 13
Glycemic load: 1

Salad with salmon

Ingredients

- **Salmon, smoked**: 100 g
- 8 leaves **Lettuce**: 40 g
- 1 **Onion**: 100 g
- 1/3 **Red pepper**: 75 g
- 1 tsp **Olive oil**: 5 g
- 1 tsp **Sunflower, seeds**: 5 g
- 1 **Cucumber**: 180 g

PREP TIME: 5 MINUTES
TOTAL TIME: 8 MINUTES

Instructions

Mix the chopped vegetables (lettuce, cucumber, onion, pepper), add the chopped smoked salmon strips, drizzle with olive oil and sprinkle with sunflower seeds.

Energy: 363 kcal
Protein: 25 g
Fat: 21 g
Carbohydrates: 19 g
Fiber: 5 g
Glycemic index: 16
Glycemic load: 2

Cod in coconut sauce

Ingredients

- **Cod, fresh**: 120 g
- 1 clove **Garlic**: 6 g
- 1/4 cup **Coconut drink**: 57 g
- 1 tsp **Olive oil**: 5 g
- 1 **Tomato**: 160 g
- 5 leaves **Lettuce**: 25 g
- 1 tsp **Paprika powder**: 4 g
- 1 tsp **Basil, dried**: 4 g
- 1 tsp **Ground turmeric**: 3 g
- 1 pinch of **black pepper**

PREP TIME: 10 MINUTES
TOTAL TIME: 30 MINUTES

Instructions

Wash the fish, dry. Cut it into pieces, sprinkle with pepper. Place it on baking foil. Prepare a marinade: pour the coconut drink into a bowl. Add turmeric, paprika and garlic squeezed through a press. Pour this marinade over the cod. Bake the fish in an oven preheated to 190 ° C for 20 minutes. Thoroughly wash the tomato, cut into cubes, and mix with basil. Serve cod accompanied by vegetables.

Energy: 327 kcal
Protein: 26 g
Fat: 19 g
Carbohydrates: 18 g
Fiber: 7 g
Glycemic index: 21
Glycemic load: 2

Tofu a'la chicken nuggets

Ingredients

PREP TIME: 15 MINUTES
TOTAL TIME: 40 MINUTES

4 portion:
- **Tofu**: 200 g
- 1 tsp **Soy sauce**: 5 g
- 1 tsp **Maple syrup**: 5 g
- 1 tsp **Taco seasoning**: 4 g
- 1 tsp **Onion powder**: 4 g
- 1/2 tsp **Paprika powder**: 2 g
- 1/2 tsp **Granulated garlic**: 2 g
- 1/2 tsp **Chicken seasoning**: 2 g

1 portion:
Energy: 88 kcal
Protein: 7 g
Fat: 4 g
Carbohydrates: 6 g
Fiber: 1 g
Glycemic index: 18
Glycemic load: 2

Instructions

To give the tofu its chicken texture place it in the freezer overnight, in the morning put it in the fridge for about 4-5 hours (this step is optional, without this step the nuggets will still be delicious). Break the drained tofu into pieces. Combine the marinade ingredients. Lightly coat the tofu with the prepared marinade. Bake the nuggets on a baking tray lined with baking paper at 180C for approx 30min until the tofu is nicely browned on the outside.

Noodles with chicken (tofu) and broccoli

PREP TIME: 5 MINUTES
TOTAL TIME: 25 MINUTES

Ingredients

- Chicken breast meat, skinless: 100 g
  (or use 1 portion of tofu nuggets)
- 1 tbsp Olive oil: 10 g
- Spaghetti pasta: 30 g
- 1/4 Broccoli: 125 g
- 1/2 Onion: 50 g
- 2 tbsp Parsley leaves: 20 g
- 1 tsp Basil, dried: 4 g
- 1 pinch of black pepper

Instructions

Preparing the chicken:
Preheat the oven to 220 ° C. Dice the meat and sprinkle
with pepper and basil. Roast the chicken for 20
minutes. Pour half of the olive oil over it.

Cook pasta according to the recipe on the package.
Halfway through cooking time, add broccoli. Finely dice
the onion. Serve chicken (tofu nuggets) with drained
pasta, broccoli, parsley, and onion. Pour the remaining
olive oil over the whole thing.

Energy: 371 kcal
Protein: 31 g
Fat: 12 g
Carbohydrates: 36 g
Fiber: 7 g
Glycemic index: 42
Glycemic load: 12

Chicken (tofu) salad with mango sauce

PREP TIME: 10 MINUTES
TOTAL TIME: 25/30 MINUTES

Ingredients

- Chicken breast meat, skinless: 100 g
  (or use 1 portion of **tofu nuggets**)
- 1/4 **Onion**: 25 g
- 1/2 **Mango**: 135 g
- 1 tbsp **Linseed oil**: 10 g
- 1 **Tomato**: 160 g
- 1 handful **Arugula**: 30 g
- 2 tbsp **Lemon juice** 12 g
- 1 pinch of **ground garlic**
- 1 pinch of **smoked paprika**
- 1 pinch of **black pepper**

Instructions

Preparing the chicken:
Preheat the oven to 220 ° C. Dice the meat and sprinkle with pepper and spices. Bake the chicken for 20 minutes.

Arrange arugula on a plate, top with meat (tofu nuggets) and tomato cut into eighths. Peel the onion, cut it into feathers, and add it to the salad.

Prepare dressing: dice mango pulp, and mix with lemon juice and olive oil to a smooth dressing.

Pour the dressing over the salad.

Energy: 339 kcal
Protein: 25 g
Fat: 12 g
Carbohydrates: 35 g
Fiber: 6 g
Glycemic index: 41
Glycemic load: 12

Chicken (tofu) and avocado salad

Ingredients

- Chicken breast meat, skinless: 100 g (or use 1 portion of **tofu nuggets**)
- 1/2 **Avocado**: 65 g
- 1/2 **Cucumber**: 90 g
- 1 tsp **Linseed oil**: 5 g
- 6 leaves **Lettuce**: 30 g
- 2 stalks of **Celery**: 90 g
- 2 tsp **Parsley, leaves**: 10 g
- 1 pinch of **garlic powder**
- 1 pinch of **black pepper**.

Instructions

Preparing the chicken:
Wash chicken meat, pat dry, and season with pepper. Fry in a skillet without additional fat.

Scoop out the avocado flesh with a spoon. Peel the celery from the fibers. Chop the parsley. Cut the garlic into small cubes. Dice the avocado, cucumber, and celery. Pour olive oil over them. Mix the vegetables with the cooled chicken (tofu nuggets).

Energy: 293 kcal
Protein: 25 g
Fat: 16 g
Carbohydrates: 13 g
Fiber: 5 g
Glycemic index: 12
Glycemic load: 1

Roasted salad with cranberries and chicken (tofu)

Ingredients

- Chicken breast meat, skinless: 100 g (or use 1 portion of **tofu nuggets**)
- 1 tbsp **Almonds flaked**: 10 g
- 2 tbsp **dried Cranberries**: 30 g
- 1 tbsp **Linseed oil**: 10 g
- 1 handful **Arugula**: 30 g
- 10 leaves **Lettuce**: 50 g
- 1 clove **Garlic**: 6 g
- 2 pinches of **dried thyme**
- 1 pinch of **black pepper**
- 1 pinch of **dried marjoram**
- 1 pinch of **dried basil**

Instructions

Preparing the chicken:
Wash, pat dry, and dice the chicken. Sprinkle with
pepper (use half the amount) and spices. Fry the
chicken in a pan without adding any fat.

Wash the lettuce, and chop it with your fingers. Peel
the garlic, squeeze it through a press, and mix it with
pepper and spices. Spread the meat (tofu nuggets) on
the plate, add the lettuce, and garlic, and sprinkle
with cranberries and roasted almonds (recipe for
roasted almonds on the next page).

Energy: 373 kcal
Protein: 26 g
Fat: 17 g
Carbohydrates: 34 g
Fiber: 5 g
Glycemic index: 12
Glycemic load: 1

Roasted almonds

Preheat the oven to 175 ° C.
Put in the oven.
Bake until golden (about 15 minutes), shaking the
baking tray from time to time.
Stir after ten minutes.

Why eat roasted almonds?

Roasted almonds without added salt or oil contain the
same nutrients as raw almonds. They are tasty and
healthy snacks.

Roasted almonds are rich in many nutrients: potassium,
phosphorus, iron, and calcium. They also contain
unsaturated fatty acids, which lower blood cholesterol
levels.

Roasted almonds are also a great source of easily
digestible vegetable protein and vitamin E, which act
as an antioxidant in the body to fight free radicals.
Vitamin E also supports the heart and circulatory
system.

Roasted almonds are also a great source of vitamins B1,
B2, B3, and fiber. These improve memory and
concentration as well as brain function.

Sandwiches with avocado paste

Ingredients

PREP TIME: 4 MINUTES
TOTAL TIME: 8 MINUTES

- 1/2 **Avocado**: 65 g
- 1 **Tomato**: 160 g
- 1 handful **Arugula**: 30 g
- 1 tsp **Parsley, leaves**: 5 g
- 2 **Radish**: 30 g
- 2 slices **Whole grain rye bread**: 60 g

Instructions

Peel the avocado. Knead with a fork until uniform. Season with your favorite spices to taste. Add the chopped tomato. Put the paste on the slices of bread. Garnish with parsley and arugula.

Energy: 291 kcal
Protein: 8 g
Fat: 12 g
Carbohydrates: 44 g
Fiber: 10 g
Glycemic index: 42
Glycemic load: 14

Peppers stuffed with quinoa and vegetables

PREP TIME: 3 MINUTES
TOTAL TIME: 18 MINUTES

Ingredients

- 1 **Red pepper**: 220 g
- 1 tsp **Parsley, leaves**: 5 g
- 1 **Tomato**: 160 g
- 2 tbsp **Pumpkin seeds**: 20 g
- 1/4 **Zucchini**: 75 g
- 2 tbsp **Quinoa**: 30 g
- 2 tbsp **Red lentils, dry seeds**: 24 g
- 1 pinch **paprika powder**
- 1 pinch **turmeric**
- 1 pinch **onion powder**
- 1 pinch **oregano**
- 1 pinch **garam masala**
- 1 pinch **black pepper**

Instructions

Cut off the top part of the pepper and remove the nest of seeds.

Boil the quinoa in water in a ratio of 1: 2.
Stew the lentils in water until it softens (or drain them from the canned pickle), then add the finely chopped zucchini to it.

Add spices (paprika powder, turmeric, onion powder, oregano, garam masala, black pepper). Set the oven to 175 ° C.

Add the chopped tomato to the lentils and zucchini. Then add the quinoa, stir, and leave it in the pot for a while (it will thicken).

Add the mixture to the hollowed-out pepper.

Put the prepared pepper into an ovenproof dish, brushed with olive oil, and placed in the oven. Bake until the pepper is golden, about 30 – 35 minutes. Garnish with parsley and pumpkin seeds.

Energy: 423 kcal
Protein: 20 g
Fat: 13 g
Carbohydrates: 62 g
Fiber: 14 g
Glycemic index: 26
Glycemic load: 12

Carrot and parsley fries with walnut and pomegranate salad

Ingredients

Fries:

- 2 **Carrots**: 100 g
- 1 **Parsley, root**: 80 g
- 1 tbsp **Linseed oil**: 10 g
- 2 pinches of **black pepper**
- 1 pinch of **dried thyme**
- 1 pinch of **dried oregano**

Salad:

- 3 **Walnuts**: 12 g
- 1 **Cucumber**: 180 g
- 1/2 **Pomegranate**: 55 g
- 1/2 clove **Garlic**: 3 g
- 1 tsp **Lemon juice**: 3 g
- 1 pinch of **paprika powder**

Instructions

Fries:
Slice the carrots and parsley into thin bars. Mix them in a bowl with half of the oil and the spices. Line a baking tray with baking paper. Arrange the vegetables and bake in a preheated to 180 ° C oven for about 30 minutes.

Salad:
Wash the cucumber, and cut it into thin slices. Put into a bowl, add chopped walnuts and pomegranate seeds, and mix. Peel and chop garlic.

Prepare dressing: in a bowl mix the other half of the oil, lemon juice, garlic, and spices.

Pour the dressing over the salad.

Energy: 331 kcal
Protein: 7 g
Fat: 19 g
Carbohydrates: 39 g
Fiber: 12 g
Glycemic index: 22
Glycemic load: 6

Celery cream soup

Ingredients

PREP TIME: 8 MINUTES
TOTAL TIME: 30 MINUTES

- 1/2 Root **Celery**: 80 g
- 1/4 Rib **Celery**: 100 g
- 1/2 cup **Canned chickpeas**: 85 g
- 3 tsp **Pumpkin, seeds**: 15 g
- 1/2 **Onion**: 50 g
- 1 tsp **Ginger, root**: 5 g
- 1 tbsp **Olive oil**: 10 g
- 1 tsp **Parsley, leaves**: 5 g
- 1 pinch of **black pepper**
- 1 cube **Vegetable cube broth**

Energy: 328 kcal
Protein: 12 g
Fat: 19 g
Carbohydrates: 30 g
Fiber: 11 g
Glycemic index: 25
Glycemic load: 5

Instructions

Heat the olive oil in a pot and sauté the chopped onion. Peel the celery, dice it, add to the onion and fry for about 4 minutes. Then add the grated ginger, pour the broth and cook for about 20 minutes, until the vegetables are tender. Mix the ready soup and season with pepper. Add drained chickpeas. Sprinkle with chopped parsley and pumpkin seeds roasted in a dry frying pan.

Lentil soup

Ingredients

PREP TIME: 10 MINUTES
TOTAL TIME: 25 MINUTES

- 4 tbsp **Red lentils, dry seeds**: 50 g
- 1/2 **Onion**: 50 g
- 3 **Mushrooms**: 60 g
- 1 cube **Vegetable cube broth**
- 1 **Carrots**: 50 g
- 1/2 **Parsley, root**: 30 g
- 1 tbsp **Olive oil**: 10 g
- 3 tbsp **Tomato paste**: 45 g
- 2 tbsp **Parsley, leaves**: 20 g
- 1 pinch of **black pepper**
- 2 pinches of **curry powder**
- 1/2 tsp **Paprika powder**: 2 g

Instructions

Dice the onion, quarter the mushrooms, fry in olive oil, and add a little water if necessary. Add spices, and mix everything. Pour the broth into the pot, add the rinsed lentils, carrots, and parsley, and cook until soft. At the end of cooking, add the tomato and tomato paste. Mix to make a cream. Garnish with chopped parsley.

Energy: 367 kcal
Protein: 19 g
Fat: 13 g
Carbohydrates: 50 g
Fiber: 13 g
Glycemic index: 27
Glycemic load: 10

Spaghetti with red lentil sauce

Ingredients

PREP TIME: 5 MINUTES
TOTAL TIME: 20 MINUTES

- Whole grain spaghetti: 30 g
- 2 tbsp **Red lentils, dry seeds**: 24 g
- 1 **Tomato**: 160 g
- 1 **Onion**: 100 g
- 1 tbsp **Linseed oil**: 10 g
- 1/2 tsp **Soy sauce**: 3 g
- 1 pinch of **paprika powder**
- 1 pinch of **dried basil**
- 1 pinch of **black pepper**

Instructions

Cook the pasta and lentils according to the instructions on the package. Dice onion and garlic and fry in oil. Put the pre-cooked and drained lentils into the pot. Add chopped tomato and spices, then blend to a smooth sauce and cook prepared in this way for about 15 minutes. Pour over the cooked pasta with the ready sauce.

Energy: 356 kcal
Protein: 15 g
Fat: 11 g
Carbohydrates: 51 g
Fiber: 7 g
Glycemic index: 35
Glycemic load: 15

Curry with tofu and eggplant

Ingredients

- **Tofu**: 90 g
- 1/2 **Eggplant**: 125 g
- 1 **Tomato**: 160 g
- 1/2 **Onion**: 50 g
- 1 tbsp **Olive oil**: 10 g
- 1 branch **Coriander**: 5 g
- 1/2 tsp **Paprika powder**: 2 g
- 1 pinch of **curry powder**
- 1 pinch of **black pepper**

Energy: 309 kcal
Protein: 15 g
Fat: 18 g
Carbohydrates: 25 g
Fiber: 7 g
Glycemic index: 19
Glycemic load: 3

PREP TIME: 10 MINUTES
TOTAL TIME: 30 MINUTES

Instructions

Peel the onion and slice it into peaks. Wash the vegetables. Cube the eggplant, tofu, and tomatoes. Brush the eggplant, tofu, and onion with olive oil. Place them on a baking tray lined with paper. Bake at 200°C until the skin of the eggplant is browned. After this time add the tomato, and season with pepper, curry, and paprika powder. Bake the whole thing for about 3-4 more minutes. Before serving sprinkle with fresh coriander.

Tortilla with salmon and hummus

Ingredients

PREP TIME: 1 MINUTES
TOTAL TIME: 3 MINUTES

- 1 **Whole grain tortilla**: 60 g
- **Salmon, smoked**: 50 g
- 1 tbsp **Hummus**: 30 g
- 1/3 **Red pepper**: 75 g
- 1 tbsp **Chives**: 5 g
- 1/4 **Cucumber**: 45 g
- 1/2 handful **Arugula**: 15 g

Instructions

Spread the tortilla with hummus, put the vegetables and smoked salmon on it. Wrap.

Energy: 373 kcal
Protein: 20 g
Fat: 16 g
Carbohydrates: 39 g
Fiber: 10 g
Glycemic index: 41
Glycemic load: 12

Pasta with green vegetables

Ingredients

- **Whole grain spaghetti**: 30 g
- 1/3 **Broccoli**: 170 g
- 1 handful ≈ 25 leaves **Fresh spinach**: 25 g
- 5 leaves **Kale**: 25 g
- 1/2 **Onion**: 50 g
- 1/2 **Zucchini**: 150 g
- 1 tbsp **Olive oil**: 10 g
- 1 pinch of **black pepper**
- 1 pinch of **paprika powder**
- 1 pinch of **dried basil**

Energy: 320 kcal
Protein: 13 g
Fat: 12 g
Carbohydrates: 42 g
Fiber: 10 g
Glycemic index: 37
Glycemic load: 13

PREP TIME: 10 MINUTES
TOTAL TIME: 35 MINUTES

Instructions

Divide the broccoli into florets and cook them in water with paprika powder and basil. Cook the pasta according to the instructions on the package. Chop the onion into small cubes. Brush the zucchini, broccoli, and onion with olive oil. Place on a baking tray lined with paper. Bake at 230°C for about 20 – 25 minutes. At the end of baking add spinach and kale. Stir the roasted vegetables into the pasta.

Spaghetti with tofu and spinach

Ingredients

- **Whole grain spaghetti**: 30 g
- **Tofu**: 90 g
- **Spinach, frozen**: 200 g
- 1 **Tomato**: 160 g
- 1 pinch of **paprika powder**
- 1 pinch of **dried basil**
- 1 pinch of **oregano**

Energy: 345 kcal
Protein: 27 g
Fat: 9 g
Carbohydrates: 42 g
Fiber: 9 g
Glycemic index: 37
Glycemic load: 12

PREP TIME: 5 MINUTES
TOTAL TIME: 20 MINUTES

Instructions

Put whole grain spaghetti on a large frying pan (if it is too long, break it in half). We add tomato, tofu, onion, frozen spinach, and favorite spices. Pour water over it and cook until the pasta is ready. If necessary, you can add more water while cooking.

Chickpea omelette

Ingredients

PREP TIME: 8 MINUTES
TOTAL TIME: 15 MINUTES

- 4 tbsp **Chickpea flour**: 48 g
- **Green peas, canned**: 100 g
- 2 tbsp **Soy milk**: 20 g
- 1/4 pieces **Red pepper**: 55 g
- 1 tbsp **Chives**: 5 g
- 1 tsp **Parsley, leaves**: 5 g
- 1 tsp **Olive oil**: 5 g
- 1 pinch of **paprika powder**
- 1 pinch of **dried oregano**
- 1 pinch of **ground turmeric**

Instructions

Pour the flour into a bowl, add spices and pour the milk, stirring with a spoon (you can use a mixer). The consistency should be quite thick. Set aside for a while and cut the vegetables during this time. Add them to the flour along with the peas. Brush the pan with olive oil and heat it up. Pour the mass into the pan and "bake" on both sides until the omelet is golden.

Energy: 331 kcal
Protein: 17 g
Fat: 8 g
Carbohydrates: 47 g
Fiber: 11 g
Glycemic index: 35
Glycemic load: 12

Caponata

Ingredients

PREP TIME: 10 MINUTES
TOTAL TIME: 25 MINUTES

- 1/2 **Eggplant**: 125 g
- 1/2 **Red pepper**: 110 g
- 1 tbsp **Olive oil**: 10 g
- 1/2 clove **Garlic**: 3 g
- 3 leaves **Fresh mint**: 3 g
- 1/2 **Onion**: 50 g
- 2 tbsp **Pistachio nuts, roasted, without salt**: 18 g
- 10 **Cashew nuts**: 20 g
- 1 **Lime**: 105 g
- 1 handful **Arugula**: 30 g
- 2 pinches of **black pepper**

Energy: 432 kcal
Protein: 12 g
Fat: 28 g
Carbohydrates: 43 g
Fiber: 12 g
Glycemic index: 17
Glycemic load: 5

Instructions

Wash and dry the pepper and eggplant. Cut the eggplants in half lengthwise. Cut the flesh in a grid. Leave the pepper whole. Lightly lubricate the vegetables with olive oil. Place the vegetables on a baking tray lined with paper and roast at 200°C until the skin is browned. Cool pepper, peel, and cut into cubes 1x1 cm. Scoop out the eggplant flesh with a spoon and chop. Add chopped garlic, spring onion, mint, and crushed nuts roasted in the oven to the chopped vegetables. Season with black pepper, and lime juice.

Quinoa curry

Ingredients

PREP TIME: 8 MINUTES
TOTAL TIME: 25 MINUTES

- 2 tbsp **Quinoa**: 28 g
- 1/4 **Onion**: 25 g
- 1/4 **Broccoli**: 125 g
- 1/2 **Carrot**: 25 g
- 1 tsp **Ginger root**: 5 g
- 1 cube **Vegetable cube broth**
- **Green peas, canned**: 150 g
- 1 **Tomato**: 160 g
- 1 clove **Garlic**: 6 g
- 2 pinches of **curry powder**
- 1 pinch of **dried hot chili pepper**
- 1 pinch of **black pepper**
- 1 pinch of **cayenne pepper**

Instructions

Dice the onion, broccoli, carrot, and ginger. Boil the quinoa in water for about 12 minutes at a ratio of 1: 2. Heat a small amount of water in a pot, add the chopped vegetables and simmer until soft, then pour in the broth, add the peas, tomato, and garlic and cook for a while. Season. At the end add milk and cook for a while. Serve with quinoa. Finally, sprinkle with parsley.

Energy: 318 kcal
Protein: 18 g
Fat: 3 g
Carbohydrates: 63 g
Fiber: 17 g
Glycemic index: 32
Glycemic load: 13

Lentil stew

Ingredients

- 3 tbsp **Lentils red, dry seeds**: 36 g
- 1/2 **Zucchini**: 150 g
- 1/4 **Leek**: 35 g
- 1 **Tomato**: 160 g
- 5 **Mushrooms**: 100 g
- 1 tbsp **Olive oil**: 10 g
- 5 leaves **Basil, fresh**: 5 g

PREP TIME: 10 MINUTES
TOTAL TIME: 25 MINUTES

Instructions

Dice the onion into small cubes, the leek into the slices, the zucchini into medium-sized pieces, and the mushrooms into quarters. Finely chop fresh basil. Heat the olive oil and fry the onion with a leek on it, add the mushrooms, and fry until released, add tomato and zucchini. Season with paprika, pour water, and mix well. Simmer all, covered, for about 5 minutes, add the lentils and mix well. Cook, covered, for 7 minutes. Sprinkle everything with fresh basil.

Energy: 300 kcal
Protein: 16 g
Fat: 12 g
Carbohydrates: 36 g
Fiber: 9 g
Glycemic index: 27
Glycemic load: 7

Tofu scrambled

Ingredients

PREP TIME: 4 MINUTES
TOTAL TIME: 8 MINUTES

- **Tofu**: 90 g
- 1 **Tomato**: 160 g
- 1/4 **Red pepper**: 55 g
- 1/2 **Onion**: 50 g
- 2 tbsp **Chives**: 10 g
- 1 tbsp **Olive oil**: 10 g
- 2 tsp **Parsley leaves**: 10 g
- 1 pinch of **curry powder**
- 1 pinch of **black pepper**
- 1 pinch of **paprika powder**

Instructions

Peel the onion, chop it finely, then let it glaze in olive oil mixed with water. When the onion is glazed, add the tofu crushed in your hands, finely chopped tomato, chopped pepper, and curry. Mix everything thoroughly and leave it on the fire for a few minutes until the tofu is tender. Add the chives, chopped parsley, stir and leave it on the fire for a while.

Energy: 307 kcal
Protein: 15 g
Fat: 18 g
Carbohydrates: 22 g
Fiber: 5 g
Glycemic index: 18
Glycemic load: 3

Quinoa with kale, broccoli and pomegranate

Ingredients

PREP TIME: 10 MINUTES
TOTAL TIME: 15 MINUTES

- 1/3 cup **Quinoa**: 60 g
- 1/4 **Broccoli**: 125 g
- 10 leaves **Kale**: 50 g
- 1/2 **Pomegranate**: 55 g
- 1/2 clove **Garlic**: 3 g
- 1 tsp **Olive oil**: 5 g
- 1 pinch of **curry powder**
- 1 pinch of **nutmeg powder**
- 1 pinch of **dried oregano**

Instructions

Pour about 1 cm of boiling water into a pot, and cook the broccoli florets in it uncovered for about 4 minutes. Then add small pieces of washed kale and cook for about 2 more minutes, stirring constantly. Pour off the remaining water, and add olive oil, pressed garlic, and spices. Keep on the heat for about 1 minute, stirring constantly. Add cooked quinoa, and mix it all up. Finally, sprinkle with pomegranate

Energy: 370 kcal
Protein: 15 g
Fat: 10 g
Carbohydrates: 60 g
Fiber: 12 g
Glycemic index: 33
Glycemic load: 16

Waffles with spinach

Ingredients

PREP TIME: 5 MINUTES
TOTAL TIME: 20 MINUTES

- 1 **Egg**
- 1/2 cup **Rye flour, type 2000**: 60 g
- 1/4 cup **Milk, 0.5% fat**: 55 g
- 1 tsp **Olive oil**: 5 g
- 1/2 tsp **Baking powder**: 2 g
- 2 handfuls **Spinach**: 50 g

Instructions

Break the egg into a bowl, and pour in the milk and oil. Add spinach and blend until smooth. Add dry ingredients: flour and baking powder. Blend again. Bake the waffles in a preheated oven.

Energy: 350 kcal
Protein: 15 g
Fat: 12 g
Carbohydrates: 49 g
Fiber: 9 g
Glycemic index: 42
Glycemic load: 17

Tabbouleh salad

Ingredients

PREP TIME: 5 MINUTES
TOTAL TIME: 10 MINUTES

- 2 tbsp **Couscous**: 26 g
- 1 **Tomato**: 160 g
- 1/4 **Cucumber**: 45 g
- 3 **Radish**: 45 g
- 1/2 clove **Garlic**: 3 g
- 1/4 **Hot chili pepper**: 5 g
- 1/2 **Onion**: 50 g
- 1 tbsp **Chives**: 5 g
- 1 tsp **Lemon juice**: 3 g
- 3 tsp **Olive oil**: 15 g
- 1 handful **Arugula**: 30 g
- 2 tsp **Parsley leaves**: 10 g

Instructions

Pour boiling water over the couscous and set aside for 5 minutes. Cucumber stripped of the seed sockets. Chop the vegetables (very finely): tomato, cucumber, radish, garlic, chili pepper, onion. Herbs chop: parsley, arugula, and chives (not necessarily finely). Season with parsley. Add the lemon juice and olive oil, and mix the ingredients thoroughly.

Energy: 309 kcal
Protein: 7 g
Fat: 15 g
Carbohydrates: 37 g
Fiber: 6 g
Glycemic index: 47
Glycemic load: 14

Salad full of power

Ingredients

PREP TIME: 5 MINUTES
TOTAL TIME: 20 MINUTES

- 2 tbsp **Buckwheat groats**: 20 g
- 1 slice **Lemon**: 12 g
- 5 leaves **Lettuce**: 25 g
- 1/2 **Avocado**: 65 g
- 1/3 **Red pepper**: 75 g
- 5 **Cherry tomatoes**: 100 g
- 1 **Egg**
- 1 tsp **Pumpkin seeds**: 5 g

Instructions

Cook groats according to the recipe on the package. Boil the egg hard. Peel and dice the avocado and drizzle with lemon juice. Dice pepper and halve tomatoes. Mix the groats with lettuce, avocado, chopped egg, pepper, and tomatoes. Sprinkle with pumpkin seeds.

Energy: 335 kcal
Protein: 14 g
Fat: 18 g
Carbohydrates: 30 g
Fiber: 6 g
Glycemic index: 34
Glycemic load: 8

Salad with quinoa, apricots, and mint

Ingredients

- 3 tbsp **Quinoa**: 42 g
- 2 **Brazil nuts**: 8 g
- 2 **Apricots**: 80 g
- 3 leaves **Fresh mint**: 3 g
- 1 **Pear**: 135 g
- **Lime peel**: 20 g
- 1 tbsp **Lime juice**: 10 g
- 2 handfuls **Spinach**: 25 g
- 1/2 tsp **Xylitol**: 3 g

PREP TIME: 5 MINUTES
TOTAL TIME: 15 MINUTES

Instructions

Cook the quinoa according to the recipe on the packet. Dice the apricots and pear, and pour over the lime juice. Mix the fruit with the mint leaves, spinach, and xylitol. Add the cooked quinoa, and sprinkle with nuts and lime zest.

Energy: 335 kcal
Protein: 10 g
Fat: 8 g
Carbohydrates: 61 g
Fiber: 9 g
Glycemic index: 31
Glycemic load: 16

Broccoli salad with dill dressing

Ingredients

- 3 **Cherry tomato**: 60 g
- 1/3 **Red pepper**: 75 g
- 1 tbsp **Lemon juice**: 6 g
- 1 tbsp **Olive oil**: 10 g
- 1 tsp **Dill**: 4 g
- 1 **Egg**
- 1/2 **Broccoli**: 250 g
- 1/2 clove **Garlic**: 3 g
- 1 pinch of **black pepper**

Energy: 288 kcal
Protein: 16 g
Fat: 16 g
Carbohydrates: 22 g
Fiber: 9 g
Glycemic index: 17
Glycemic load: 2

PREP TIME: 5 MINUTES
TOTAL TIME: 15 MINUTES

Instructions

Wash broccoli, divide it into florets, and cook (preferably half hard, it is important not to overcook). Hard boil the egg, peel, and cut into eighths. Wash peppers and cut them into thin strips. Wash tomatoes and cut them in half. Prepare dressing from olive oil, lemon juice, pepper, and crushed garlic (you can omit it if you don't like it). In a container arrange the broccoli florets, peppers, tomatoes, and egg pieces. Pour the dressing over the salad just before eating.

Salad with corn, pepper and chia seeds

Ingredients

PREP TIME: 5 MINUTES
TOTAL TIME: 5 MINUTES

- 3 tbsp **Canned Corn**: 45 g
- 1 tbsp **Olive oil**: 10 g
- 1/3 **Red pepper**: 75 g
- 1 **Tomato**: 160 g
- 8 leaves **Lettuce**: 40 g
- 1 tbsp **Chia seeds**: 10 g
- 1 pinch of **black pepper**
- 1 slice **Wholemeal bread**: 30 g

Instructions

Chop the vegetables. Grind the chia seeds. Stir in the olive oil and season to taste. Serve with a slice of bread.

Energy: 315 kcal
Protein: 7 g
Fat: 15 g
Carbohydrates: 43 g
Fiber: 11 g
Glycemic index: 41
Glycemic load: 14

Salad with nuts, avocado dressing and wholemeal bread

Ingredients

- 1/2 **Avocado**: 65 g
- 1 clove **Garlic**: 6 g
- 2 leaves **Chinese cabbage**: 100 g
- 2 tsp **Dill**: 8 g
- 1 tbsp **Hazelnuts**: 15 g
- 1/2 **Red pepper**: 110 g
- 3 **Radish**: 45 g
- 1 slice **Wholemeal bread**: 30 g

Energy: 348 kcal
Protein: 10 g
Fat: 20 g
Carbohydrates: 38 g
Fiber: 12 g
Glycemic index: 33
Glycemic load: 8

PREP TIME: 5 MINUTES
TOTAL TIME: 5 MINUTES

Instructions

Mash the ripe avocado with a fork together with the squeezed one press with garlic and spices to taste. Slice the ingredients. Mix everything. Serve with bread.

Quinoa salad with vegetables

Ingredients

PREP TIME: 5 MINUTES
TOTAL TIME: 20 MINUTES

- 3 tbsp **Quinoa**: 42 g
- 1 tbsp **Olive oil**: 10 g
- 1 **Cucumber**: 180 g
- 1/4 **Red pepper**: 55 g
- 2 leaves **Chinese cabbage**: 100 g
- 1 tbsp **Lemon juice**: 6 g
- 1 tbsp **Mustard**: 20 g
- 1 clove **Garlic**: 6 g
- 3 **Radish**: 45 g
- 1 tbsp **Lentils, sprouts**: 10 g
- 1 tsp **Parsley, leaves**: 5 g
- 1 pinch of **black pepper**

Instructions

Rinse quinoa thoroughly, pour boiling water over it and cook for about 15 minutes, stirring occasionally. Slice the remaining ingredients and mix with the cooked groats. Season to taste. Mix the oil, lemon juice, and mustard, and then mix with the salad. Garnish with lentil sprouts and parsley.

Energy: 354 kcal
Protein: 11 g
Fat: 14 g
Carbohydrates: 49 g
Fiber: 9 g
Glycemic index: 29
Glycemic load: 11

Salad with lamb's lettuce

Ingredients

- 1 handful **Lamb's lettuce**: 25 g
- 3 tbsp **Canned red bean**: 90 g
- 3 tbsp **Canned green peas**: 50 g
- 3 tbsp **Canned corn**: 45 g
- 2 tsp **Dill**: 8 g
- 1 tsp **Linseed oil**: 5 g
- 4 **Green olives**: 12 g
- 4 **Cherry tomato**: 80 g
- 1 pinch of **black pepper**

Instructions

Drain the beans, peas, and corn from the pickle. Dill the dill, lamb's lettuce, olives, and cherry tomatoes. Mix all. Mix the olive oil with spices. Pour salad dressing.

Energy: 280 kcal
Protein: 12 g
Fat: 9 g
Carbohydrates: 41 g
Fiber: 10 g
Glycemic index: 48
Glycemic load: 15

Rocket salad

Ingredients

- 2 handfuls **Arugula**: 60 g
- 1 tbsp **Linseed oil**: 10 g
- 5 **Cherry tomato**: 100 g
- 2 tbsp **Sunflower seeds**: 20 g

PREP TIME: 5 MINUTES
TOTAL TIME: 10 MINUTES

Instructions

Wash and dry the cherry tomatoes and rocket. Roast the sunflower seeds for 3 minutes in a dry frying pan. Put the previously ground and washed ingredients into the bowl and mix them with the roasted sunflower seeds. Finally, pour a spoon of oil over it.

Energy: 238 kcal
Protein: 7 g
Fat: 19 g
Carbohydrates: 11 g
Fiber: 3 g
Glycemic index: 30
Glycemic load: 2

Smoothie with avocado and fruit

Ingredients

PREP TIME: 2 MINUTES
TOTAL TIME: 5 MINUTES

- 1/2 **Banana**: 65 g
- 1/2 **Avocado**: 65 g
- 5 tbsp **Coconut drink**: 50 g
- 1 **Orange**: 240 g
- 1/3 cup **Water**: 80 g
- **Sweetener**: as desired

Instructions

Blend all ingredients.

Energy: 295 kcal
Protein: 4 g
Fat: 11 g
Carbohydrates: 48 g
Fiber: 8 g
Glycemic index: 40
Glycemic load: 16

Bounty cocktail

Ingredients

PREP TIME: 2 MINUTES
TOTAL TIME: 4 MINUTES

- 1 **Banana**: 130 g
- 1 tbsp **Coconut shredded**: 6 g
- 1 tbsp **Linseed**: 10 g
- 2 cubes **Dark chocolate**: 12 g
- 2 tbsp **Coconut drink**: 20 g
- **Sweetener**: as desired

Instructions

Blend all ingredients.

Energy: 284 kcal
Protein: 5 g
Fat: 11 g
Carbohydrates: 43 g
Fiber: 6 g
Glycemic index: 52
Glycemic load: 17

Green cocktail

Ingredients

PREP TIME: 3 MINUTES
TOTAL TIME: 6 MINUTES

- 1/3 cup **Coconut drink**: 80 g
- 1/3 cup **Water**: 80 g
- 5 leaves **Basil, fresh**: 5 g
- 1 **Kiwi**: 80 g
- 1 **Green banana**: 130 g
- 5 **Cashews**: 10 g
- 1 **Lime**: 105 g
- **Sweetener**: as desired

Instructions

Peel the fruit and blend it with the remaining ingredients for a smoothie.

Energy: 278 kcal
Protein: 5 g
Fat: 6 g
Carbohydrates: 58 g
Fiber: 7 g
Glycemic index: 41
Glycemic load: 14

Cocoa waffles

Ingredients

- **Flax egg**:
  1 tbsp **linseed**: 10 g
  + 3 tbsp **water**: 30 g
- 1/3 cup **Buckwheat flakes**:
  35 g
- 1 tsp **Cocoa**: 5 g
- 1 tsp **Xylitol**: 6 g
- 2 tsp **Peanut butter**: 20 g
- 2 tbsp **Sparkling water**:
  20 g

PREP TIME: 10 MINUTES
TOTAL TIME: 18 MINUTES

Instructions

Mix one tablespoon of
ground flaxseed with three
tablespoons of water. Add
sparkling water and
xylitol, and mix to a
liquid form. Add buckwheat
flakes and cocoa. Stir
again. Pour the mass into
the waffle iron. Bake
waffles. Brush the
finished waffles with
peanut butter.

Energy: 326 kcal
Protein: 12 g
Fat: 15 g
Carbohydrates: 43 g
Fiber: 7 g
Glycemic index: 45
Glycemic load: 13

Yoghurt and Blueberries dessert

Ingredients

- 2 **Grain biscuits**: 10 g
- **Natural soy yogurt**: 200 g
- **Blueberries**: 200 g
- 1 tsp **Xylitol**: 6 g

PREP TIME: 5 MINUTES
TOTAL TIME: 10 MINUTES

Instructions

Place the whole grain biscuits at the bottom of the glass. Blend chilled yogurt with xylitol. Pour half the weight over the biscuits. Arrange half a serving of blackberries. Pour in the second half of the yogurt mass. Place the second part of the blackberries on top.

Energy: 273 kcal
Protein: 10 g
Fat: 6 g
Carbohydrates: 47 g
Fiber: 7 g
Glycemic index: 33
Glycemic load: 11

Quinoa with raspberries

Ingredients

PREP TIME: 3 MINUTES
TOTAL TIME: 18 MINUTES

- 4 tbsp **Quinoa**: 56 g
- 1/2 cup **Raspberries**: 65 g
- 1 cup **Soy milk**: 240 g
- 1 tbsp **Almonds**: 10 g
- 1 pinch of **cinnamon powder**
- 1/2 tsp **Xylitol**: 3 g

Instructions

Cook the quinoa according to the recipe on the package. Add milk, cinnamon, and xylitol to it. Sprinkle with fruit and almond.

Energy: 429 kcal
Protein: 20 g
Fat: 16 g
Carbohydrates: 55 g
Fiber: 12 g
Glycemic index: 29
Glycemic load: 12

Bounty balls

Ingredients

PREP TIME: 5 MINUTES
TOTAL TIME: 20 MINUTES

- 4 tbsp **Coconut shredded**: 24 g
- 6 cubes **Dark chocolate, 70-85% cocoa**: 36 g
- 3 tbsp **Water**: 30 g
- 3 tbsp **Coconut drink**: 30 g
- 1/2 tsp **Xylitol**: 3 g

Instructions

Boil the milk with 3 tablespoons of water. After a while, add the shavings, cook, and stir until the shavings soak up the liquid. Leave to cool down. Form oblong bars from the mass and place them on the baking tray. Melt the chocolate and pour it over the cooled coconut bars. Leave it to cool down completely.

Energy: 384 kcal
Protein: 4 g
Fat: 31 g
Carbohydrates: 26 g
Fiber: 9 g
Glycemic index: 25
Glycemic load: 4

Cherry-nut cake

Ingredients

PREP TIME: 15 MINUTES
TOTAL TIME: 50 MINUTES

- **Flax egg**:
  4 tbsp **linseed**: 40 g
  + 12 tbsp **water**: 120 g
- 1/2 cup **Buckwheat flour**:
  70 g
- 1/4 cup **Coconut flour**:
  30 g
- 1 tsp **Baking powder**: 4 g
- **Frozen cherries**: 200 g
- 8 **Walnuts**: 32 g
- 1 tsp **Xylitol**: 6 g

Instructions

Mix four tablespoons of ground flaxseed with twelve tablespoons of water. Add xylitol and mix. Sift into the flour mass and mix. Pour the dough into a mold. Place the cherries on top and bake the cake at 180 ° C for 35 minutes. At the end of baking, add the crushed walnuts on top.

The whole cake:
Energy: 876 kcal
Protein: 31 g
Fat: 38 g
Carbohydrates: 119 g
Fiber: 28 g
Glycemic index: 24
Glycemic load: 16

Muffins with apples and cinnamon

Ingredients

PREP TIME: 10-15
MINUTES
TOTAL TIME: 40-45
MINUTES

- 1 Egg
  (or **Flax egg**:
  1 tbsp **linseed**: 10 g
  + 3 tbsp **water**: 30 g)
- 1/2 cup **Coconut drink**:
  120 g
- 3 tbsp **Chickpea flour**:
  36 g
- 1 tsp **Olive oil**: 5 g
- 1/2 tsp **Xylitol**: 3 g
- 1/2 **Apple**: 80 g
- 1 pinch of **cinnamon
  powder**

Instructions

Break the eggs (in the
vegan version, prepare a
flax egg: Mix one
tablespoons of ground
flaxseed with three
tablespoons of water), add
sparkling water and
coconut drink, and mix.
Add flour, xylitol, and
cinnamon to the mass and
mix again until it is
liquid. Peel the apple and
slice it. Add to the
dough. Brush the molds
with olive oil. Transfer
the mass. Bake at 180 ° C
for 30 minutes until the
stick is dry.

Energy: 334 kcal
Protein: 15 g
Fat: 14 g
Carbohydrates: 37 g
Fiber: 6 g
Glycemic index: 35
Glycemic load: 9

Apple with crumble

Ingredients

PREP TIME: 5 MINUTES
TOTAL TIME: 30 MINUTES

- 1 **Apple**: 160 g
- 2 tbsp **Chickpea flour**: 24 g
- 1 tbsp **Linseed oil**: 10 g
- 2 pinches of **cinnamon powder**
- **Sweetener**: as desired

Instructions

Preheat the oven to 200 ° C. To prepare the crumble: in a bowl, mix the dry ingredients (including the sweetener). Add oil and mix all together. Slice the apples and place them in a baking pan lined with baking paper. Sprinkle the apples with the prepared crumble. Bake the whole thing for about 25 minutes.

Energy: 267 kcal
Protein: 6 g
Fat: 12 g
Carbohydrates: 34 g
Fiber: 7 g
Glycemic index: 43
Glycemic load: 12

Coconut pineapple chia pudding

Ingredients

PREP TIME: 10 MINUTES
TOTAL TIME: 40 MINUTES

- 1/2 cup **Coconut drink**: 120 g
- 1/4 cup **Coconut milk**: 55 g
- 3 tsp **Chia seeds**: 15 g
- 2 slices **Pineapple**: 80 g
- 1 pinch of **cinnamon powder**
- 1/2 tsp **Xylitol**: 3 g

Instructions

Mix the coconut milk with the coconut drink, then add the chia, cinnamon, and xylitol. Mix it all together. Set aside in the fridge for 30 minutes to swell or preferably overnight. Stir a few times in the meantime. Blend the fresh pineapple slices into a mousse, and pour over the milk pudding. Garnish with a slice of pineapple and a pinch of cinnamon.

Energy: 251 kcal
Protein: 4 g
Fat: 17 g
Carbohydrates: 22 g
Fiber: 6 g
Glycemic index: 41
Glycemic load: 6

Almond coconut pralines

Ingredients

PREP TIME: 5 MINUTES
TOTAL TIME: 15 MINUTES

- 1/2 cup **Almond flour**: 55 g
- 1 tbsp **Coconut shredded**: 6 g
- 1/2 tsp **Lemon juice**: 2 g
- 1 tsp **Linseed oil**: 5 g
- 1 tsp **Honey**: 12 g

Instructions

Put almond flour in a bowl, add honey and slightly heated oil, and mix by hand, knead and – pressing firmly – form balls. You can also add half a teaspoon of lemon juice to break the sweetness. Coat in coconut shredded.

Energy: 441 kcal
Protein: 12 g
Fat: 36 g
Carbohydrates: 23 g
Fiber: 8 g
Glycemic index: 54
Glycemic load: 8

Blueberry porridge with linseed and cinnamon

Ingredients

- 4 tbsp **Oatmeal**: 40 g
- 3 tbsp **Blueberries**: 45 g
- 2 tbsp **Soybean yogurt**: 40 g
- 1 tsp **Cocoa**: 5 g
- 1 tbsp **Linseed**: 10 g
- 1 pinch of **cinnamon powder**
- 1/2 tsp **Xylitol**: 3 g

Energy: 269 kcal
Protein: 10 g
Fat: 8 g
Carbohydrates: 41 g
Fiber: 8 g
Glycemic index: 48
Glycemic load: 15

PREP TIME: 5 MINUTES
TOTAL TIME: 10 MINUTES

Instructions

Put the oat flakes in a bowl, pour a small amount of boiling water over them, cover and wait for the flakes to absorb the water. Mix the oat flakes with the yoghurt and xylitol. Sprinkle with cinnamon and cocoa. Grind the flaxseed in a grinder and sprinkle over the oatmeal. Add the blueberries.

*Contrary to popular belief, **porridge** that is not overcooked is an example of a moderate glycemic load meal that is ideal for women with PCOS. In the context of insulin resistance occurring in PCOS, it is a very good option e.g. breakfast. Increased insulin sensitivity will result in a reduced testosterone concentration, and thus a better picture of PCOS (minimizing hirsutism, increasing the regularity of menstrual cycles). When it comes to insulin sensitivity, one cannot but mention cinnamon, which increases the sensitivity of cells to insulin. A beneficial product in polycystic ovary syndrome is also **linseed** – a rich source of anti-inflammatory omega-3 acids. It is definitely better to add them freshly ground because that's when we can "extract" the essence of these beans.*

3-DAYS MENU 1800 KCAL

1 DAY

Energy: 1794 kcal
Protein: g Fat: 94 g Carbohydrates: 177 g

Breakfast: **Super bowl**

- 1/2 **Apple**: 80 g
- 5 **Walnuts**: 20 g
- 1/3 cup **Coconut drink**: 80 g
- 2 tbsp **Quinoa, seeds**: 28 g
- 3 tbsp **Sunflower seeds, shelled**: 15 g
- 3 tbsp **Blueberries**: 45 g
- 1-2 tsp **Sweetener**

Cook the quinoa in coconut drink with the sweetener. Put the quinoa into a bowl, and put some fruit and nuts next to it. Sprinkle with sunflower seeds.

Energy: 402 kcal
Protein: 11 g Fat: 21 g Carbohydrates: 44 g

Snack: **Salad with sesame & sunflower**

- 1 tbsp **Linseed oil**: 10 g
- 6 **Cherry tomato**: 120 g
- 2 tsp **Sesame, seeds**: 10 g
- 3 tsp **Sunflower seeds shelled**: 15 g
- 1 handful **Spinach**: 25 g
- 1 tbsp **Lemon juice**: 6 g

Cut cherry tomatoes in half. In a dry pan roast sunflower seeds and sesame seeds. Mix all ingredients in one bowl, drizzle with lemon juice, and sprinkle with roasted seeds. Drizzle with linseed oil.

Energy: 271 kcal
Protein: 8 g Fat: 23 g Carbohydrates: 10 g

Lunch: **Chicken with asparagus and buckwheat**

- **Chicken breast meat, skinless**: 120 g
- 3 tbsp **Buckwheat groats**: 40 g
- 1/2 clove **Garlic**: 3 g
- 6 **Asparagus**: 180 g
- 1 tsp **Dill**: 5 g
- 2 tsp **Pumpkin, seeded, shelled**: 10 g
- 1 tbsp **Olive oil**: 10 g
- 2 tsp **Parsley**: 10 g
- 1 pinch of **dried basil**
- 1 pinch of **black pepper**
- 1 pinch of **paprika powder**

Preheat the oven to 220 degrees. Sprinkle the chicken with pepper and paprika powder. Wash the asparagus, and break off the hard ends (they will break by themselves in the right place). Place asparagus on each piece of breast and roll up the fillets. Add pressed garlic, chopped dill, and basil. Drizzle with olive oil and bake uncovered for 15 minutes before placing in the oven. Cook the groats according to the recipe on the package. Put everything on a plate, and serve with pumpkin seeds.

Energy: 469 kcal
Protein: 39 g Fat: 18 g Carbohydrates: 42 g

Snack: **Chia pudding**

- 4 tbsp **Chia seeds**: 40 g
- 4 tbsp **Blueberries**: 60 g
- 1 cup **Coconut drink**: 240 g

Pour the coconut drink into a glass, add the chia seeds, and stir vigorously. Put in the fridge for a few hours for the seeds to swell. Pour finished chia into a bowl, and top with berries.

Energy: 276 kcal
Protein: 7 g Fat: 14 g Carbohydrates: 32 g

Dinner: **Sandwiches with hummus**

- 2 slices **Wholemeal rye bread**: 60 g
- 3 tbsp **Hummus**: 90 g
- 5 leaves **Lettuce**: 25 g
- 1/2 **Cucumber**: 90 g
- 1 tbsp **Chives**: 5 g
- 1 tbsp **Radish, sprouts**: 10 g
- 1 pinch of **black pepper**

Spread hummus on the bread. Place lettuce and cucumber slices on sandwiches. Sprinkle with chopped chives, pepper, and radish sprouts.

Energy: 375 kcal
Protein: 12 g Fat: 17 g Carbohydrates: 48 g

2 DAY

Energy: 1802 kcal
Protein: 77 g Fat: 82 g Carbohydrates: 219 g

Breakfast: **Raspberry Oatmeal**

- 3 tbsp **Oatmeal**: 30 g
- 1 cup **Coconut drink**: 240 g
- 1 cup **Raspberries**: 30 g
- 2 pinches of **cinnamon**
- **Sweetener**: as desired

Boil oatmeal, sweetener, and cinnamon in coconut drink and bring to a boil, stirring frequently. Let stand covered for about 5 minutes. Serve with raspberries.

Energy: 223 kcal
Protein: 6 g Fat: 5 g Carbohydrates: 45 g

Snack: **Tuna, avocado, and sun-dried tomato sandwiches**

- 2 slices **Wholemeal rye bread**: 60 g
- 4 tbsp **Tuna in own sauce (in water)**: 120 g
- 1/3 **Avocado**: 45 g
- 4 slices **Tomato**: 80 g
- 1 tsp **Parsley**: 5 g
- 1 pinch of **black pepper**
- 1 pinch of **dried oregano**

Drain the fish from the marinade. Cut the tomatoes into slices. Cut avocado in half, scoop out the flesh, and mash with a fork. Wash and chop parsley. Put all ingredients (except tomato) into a bowl and mix thoroughly. Slice the bread, spread the paste, and place the tomato on the sandwich.

Energy: 349 kcal
Protein: 30 g Fat: 10 g Carbohydrates: 39 g

Lunch: **Curry with tofu, nuts, and coconut milk**

- **Tofu**: 100 g
- 3 **Mushrooms:** 60 g
- 1/4 **Onion**: 25 g
- 1/2 cup **Coconut milk**: 120 g
- **Green beans, frozen**: 80 g
- 1/3 **Red pepper**: 75 g
- 2 **Walnuts**: 8 g
- 1/2 tsp **Soy sauce**: 3 g
- 1/2 tsp **Lemon juice**: 2 g
- 2 tsp **Parsley**: 10 g
- 1 pinch of **ground turmeric**
- 1 pinch of **curry powder**
- 1 pinch of **black pepper**
- 1 pinch of **paprika powder**

Dice the tofu, slice the mushrooms and peppers, and dice the onion. Heat up some coconut milk in a pot or a large frying pan, and throw the onions and peppers into it. Stew for a few minutes. Then add curry powder and chopped tofu. Stew for another 2-3 minutes. Add the mushrooms, green beans, remaining coconut milk, curry powder, turmeric, black pepper, and sweet paprika. Stew for 10-15 minutes until vegetables are soft. In a pan roast nut (without adding fat). Drizzle with lemon juice and sprinkle with parsley.

Energy: 491 kcal
Protein: 21 g Fat: 35 g Carbohydrates: 28 g

Snack: **Hazelnut-chocolate mousse with fruits**

- 1/2 **Banana**: 65 g
- 1/4 **Avocado**: 34 g
- 1/2 tsp **Cocoa**: 3 g
- 6 tbsp **Blueberries**: 90 g
- 1 cup **Raspberries**: 130 g
- 4 **Brazil nuts**: 16 g
- **Sweetener**: as desired

Peel and slice the banana. (Be sure to choose less ripe bananas). Scoop out the flesh from the avocado. Crush the nuts. Blend all ingredients together. Add sweetener as desired. Eat mousse with fruit.

Energy: 361 kcal
Protein: 7 g Fat: 17 g Carbohydrates: 53 g

Dinner: **Salad with buckwheat, chickpeas, and carrots**

- 2 tbsp **Buckwheat groats**: 40 g
- 5 tbsp **Chickpeas:** 100 g
- 1 **Carrot**: 50 g
- 1 handful **Spinach**: 25 g
- 1/2 **Onion**: 50 g
- 2 tbsp **Chives**: 10 g
- 1 tbsp **Olive oil**: 10 g
- 4 **Black olives**: 12 g
- 1/2 tsp **Paprika powder**: 2 g
- 1 tsp **Basil, dried**: 4 g
- 1 pinch of **dried chili peppers**
- 1 pinch of **coriander**

Cook buckwheat in water with paprika powder and basil. Drain the canned chickpeas and rinse under running water. Wash, peel, and cut the carrots into posts. Peel the onion and cut it into peaks. Prepare a dressing by mixing olive oil with chopped chives. Put the ingredients on a plate and pour the dressing over them. Mix all together and sprinkle with chopped coriander.

Energy: 377 kcal
Protein: 12 g Fat: 15 g Carbohydrates: 52 g

3 DAY

Energy: 1799 kcal
Protein: 78 g Fat: 87 g Carbohydrates: 194 g

Breakfast: **Cocoa porridge**

- 3 tbsp **Oatmeal**: 30 g
- 3 tbsp **Blueberries**: 45 g
- 1 tsp **Cocoa**: 5 g
- 3 **Walnuts**: 12 g
- 1 tbsp **Chia seeds**: 10 g
- 1 cup **Almond drink**: 240 g
- 3 pinches of **cinnamon powder**

Boil oatmeal, cocoa, cinnamon, and chia seeds in milk, and bring the whole thing to a boil while stirring frequently. Set aside for about 5 minutes, covered. Serve with blueberries and nuts.

Energy: 353 kcal
Protein: 10 g Fat: 16 g Carbohydrates: 45 g

Snack: **Red sandwich with sprouts**

- 2 slices **Wholemeal rye bread**: 60 g
- 1 **Red pepper**: 220 g
- 1 **Tomato**: 160 g
- 1 tbsp **Lemon juice**: 6 g
- 1 tsp **Parsley, leaves**: 5 g
- 1 tsp **Radish, sprouts:** 10 g

Dice pepper and tomato and mix with parsley and lemon juice. Place the paste on the bread. Decorate with sprouts.

Energy: 245 kcal
Protein: 8 g Fat: 2 g Carbohydrates: 52 g

Lunch: **Trout with quinoa and vegetables**

- 2 tbsp **Quinoa, seed**: 28 g
- **Trout, fresh**: 120 g
- 1 tbsp **Olive oil**: 10 g
- 3 slices **Lemon**: 36 g
- **Green beans, frozen:** 100 g
- 1 tsp **Radish, sprouts**: 10 g
- 1/2 tsp **Paprika powder**: 2 g
- 1 pinch of **black pepper**
- 1 pinch of **dried basil**
- 1 pinch of **ground turmeric**
- 1 pinch of **dried thyme**

Rub the fish with olive oil, and pepper. Put thyme sprigs and lemon inside the fish. Bake for about 30 minutes at 190 degrees. Cook quinoa and green beans according to the recipe on the package (addition of salt replace the spices). Serve with sprouts.

Energy: 445 kcal
Protein: 30 g Fat: 23 g Carbohydrates: 31 g

Snack: **Amaranth with apple and cinnamon**

- 3 tbsp **Amaranth, grain**: 36 g
- 1/2 **Apple**: 80 g
- 2/3 cup **Almond drink**: 180 g
- 5 **Walnuts**: 20 g
- 1 pinch of **cinnamon powder**

Rinse amaranth grains underwater and then roast in a pan (without adding fat) to get rid of the characteristic bitterness. Pour vegetable beverage over grains and cook over low heat for about 15 minutes, stirring from time to time. Peel and grate the apple and mix with cinnamon. Put cooked amaranth into a bowl, and add apple and crushed nuts.

Energy: 360 kcal
Protein: 10 g Fat: 17 g Carbohydrates: 45 g

Dinner: **Salad with egg and vegetables**

- 5 leaves **Lettuce**: 25 g
- 1 **Tomato**: 160 g
- 1/2 **Cucumber**: 90 g
- 2 **Eggs**
- 1/3 **Avocado**: 45 g
- 1 tsp **Olive oil**: 5 g
- 2 tsp **Pumpkin, seeded, shelled**: 10 g
- 1 pinch of **black pepper**
- 1 pinch of **ground turmeric**
- 1 tsp **Basil, dried**: 4 g

Boil the eggs. Rinse lettuce, and transfer to a plate. Slice the tomato, avocado, and cucumber and put them on the lettuce. Season and top with olive oil.

Energy: 395 kcal
Protein: 20 g Fat: 27 g Carbohydrates: 19 g

Printed in Great Britain
by Amazon

44727417R00066